Public Opi
about Abortion

SECOND EDITION

Public Opinion about Abortion

Everett Carll Ladd
and
Karlyn H. Bowman

The AEI Press

Publisher for the American Enterprise Institute

WASHINGTON, D.C.

1999

ISBN 0-8447-7126-0

1   3   5   7   9   10   8   6   4   2

THE AEI PRESS
Publisher for the American Enterprise Institute
1150 Seventeenth Street, N.W.
Washington, D.C. 20036

Contents

Acknowledgments

The authors would like to thank Melissa Knauer of AEI for the many hours she spent scouring the files for questions included here and proofreading these numbers against original survey releases. Her attention to detail is greatly valued. Rob Persons of the Roper Center ran data for inclusion and helped us fill in some of the blanks on the original manuscript. Lisa Ferraro Parmalee, also of the Roper Center, read the manuscript and provided very useful suggestions about its content and tone. AEI's crack team of editors always improves our prose. In this instance the credit goes to Cheryl Weissman, who has a gift for finding just the right word as well as a talent for adroit editing. AEI interns Sara Owen and Nathan Gragg also helped at every stage.

Public Opinion about Abortion

N ineteen ninety-eight marked the twenty-fifth anniversary of one of the most controversial decisions in the history of the Supreme Court. *Roe v. Wade* and subsequent Court decisions have not settled the abortion issue for pro-life and pro-choice activists. The vast majority of Americans, however, have rendered a clear judgment.

Public opinion on abortion has been remarkably stable over the past quarter century, as the data in this monograph show. These findings undermine the commonly held view that public opinion is fickle and changeable. Although it is unlikely that many people have read the Supreme Court decisions on abortion, Americans understand the issues the Court has addressed. Moreover, they are clear as to what they believe abortion policy should be. On questions that have been repeated many times, opinion barely moves. None of the Court decisions after *Roe v. Wade* has altered the basic configuration of attitudes on abortion.

Opinion about abortion is stable, but it is certainly not one-dimensional. Some questions pull people in one direction, others draw them in another. Opinion is not only clear; it is also complex. Survey researchers have explored the nuances in opinion thoroughly and regularly, and the polls provide a unique perspective on the issue.

We have grouped the major questions about abortion into six areas. We begin by looking at a handful of questions that stress the sanctity of life. The second group of questions emphasizes the importance of individual choice. Next, we look at public views about the circumstances under which abortion should be permitted, and then at people's views about what abortion policy should be. Following this, we explore the views of different groups in the population about abortion. The final group of questions looks at abortion as an election issue. The national polls help us to understand how important the abortion issue is to voters, and exit polls of voters as they leave their voting booths provide deeper insights into the political power of the issue. Although we refer in the text to questions that have been asked only once or twice, the tables for the most part present trends.

The Sanctity of Life and the Importance of Choice

In April 1973, three months after the Supreme Court's *Roe v. Wade* decision, Louis Harris and Associates asked people whether they tended to agree or disagree with some provocative statements about permitting abortion in the first three months of pregnancy.[1] Sixty-three percent said they tended to agree with the statement "It's against God's will to destroy any human life, especially that of an unborn baby," and 28 percent tended to disagree. Another statement was phrased this way: "So long as a doctor has to be consulted, the matter of an abortion is only a question of a woman's decision with her doctor's professional advice." Sixty-eight percent tended to agree with this statement, and 23 percent tended to disagree.

These two questions illustrate a deep tension in public

---

1. In several of its survey questions, Louis Harris and Associates refers to the Supreme Court decision in *Roe v. Wade* as involving the first three months of pregnancy. The Court decision does this, of course, but it is much broader. Writing in *Public Opinion Quarterly* in 1978, Ray Adamek calls the Harris phrasing "curious and misleading." "It is misleading," he says, "because, although accurate as far as it goes, it tends to give those uninformed about the [Roe] decision the impression that the Court did not legalize abortion after three months." Adamek suggests that although the phrasing measures opinion on a part of the Court's decision, it does not measure opinion about the full decision.

opinion on abortion. People recognize that human life is precious, and they think it should be protected. At the same time, they feel strongly that individual choice should be respected. Questions tapping both these core sentiments pull the public in different directions. Most Americans are at once pro-choice and pro-life.

The pollsters have posed many different questions exploring fundamental views about life. A number of them ask whether abortion is murder. Large numbers of respondents consistently say that it is. Table 1 presents the results from a question CBS News and the *New York Times* began asking sixteen years ago. (Tables follow the text, beginning on page 19.) In 1983, 57 percent said that abortion is "the same thing as murdering a child," while 30 percent said that "abortion is not murder because a fetus isn't a person." The four askings of this version of the CBS News/*New York Times* question produced majority support for the view that abortion is murder. Wording can affect responses, of course. The news organizations changed the wording of the second half of the question in 1989 to "abortion is not murder because the fetus really isn't a child," and the responses have moved slightly. In the most recent iteration of the question in January 1998, 50 percent said abortion was the same thing as murdering a child, but 38 percent disagreed.

In July 1989, CBS News/*New York Times* interviewers asked those people who said that abortion was the same thing as murdering a child (40 percent of the sample) whether they believed this was still the case in the first three months of pregnancy. Over 90 percent said that it was.

Other survey questions exploring the belief that abortion is murder produce somewhat different results, depending on how questions are worded and how surveys are designed and constructed. All find considerable support for this judgment. A March 1989 *Los Angeles Times* poll devoted almost entirely to the abortion issue found a slightly higher percentage (58 percent) than the early CBS News/*New York Times* polls agreeing with the statement "Abortion is murder." Forty-two percent of the 58 percent agreed strongly. Thirty-four percent disagreed, 19 percent strongly. The *Los Angeles Times* survey included a question that asked whether life "begins at conception, or at birth, or somewhere in between." A plurality (41 percent) chose conception, 27 percent said somewhere in between, and 15 percent said it began at birth. The *Los Angeles Times* has not repeated this question.

A question posed in the 1996 Survey of American Political Culture (a Gallup Organization/University of Virginia project) found 38 percent agreeing with the statement "Abortion is just as bad as killing a person who has already been born—it is murder." Ten percent agreed that "abortion is murder, but it is not as bad as killing someone who has already been born," and 26 percent agreed with the statement "Abortion is not murder, but it does involve the taking of a human life." Only 16 percent chose the position "Abortion is not murder—it is a surgical procedure for removing human tissue." A question asked in 1994 and 1995 by Yankelovich Partners in its survey work for *Time* and CNN and by Gallup in 1998 (in its work for CNN and *USA Today*) reinforces the findings above. In 1998, 48 percent described abortion as an act of murder, and 45 percent did not feel that way (table 2).

Other questions reveal people's deep personal reservations about abortion, and these, no doubt, contribute to views about what abortion policy should be. A Gallup question posed for CNN and *USA Today* in 1995 found that 51 percent called abortion morally wrong, but 34 percent did not. Two questions asked in 1996 Opinion Dynamics polls for Fox News found pluralities saying that they were personally against abortion (table 3). A question in the Gallup/University of Virginia survey mentioned above asks a large national sample about various actions. The introduction to the question begins: "How wrong do you personally think it is when people engage in the following behavior?" One of the actions is "abortion during the first three months of pregnancy." Thirty-four percent said this was "wrong for all, and should not be legally tolerated," 16 percent "wrong for all, but should be tolerated," 24 percent "right for some, but not for me personally," 6 percent "right for me, but not necessarily for others," and 11 percent "right for all." Eight percent responded by saying that this was "not a moral issue." A Roper Starch Worldwide question found identical near majorities in 1992 and in 1995, saying that the bad effects outweighed the good ones in abortion (table 4).

Belief in the sanctity of life is a conviction that influences attitudes about abortion policy.

The Significance of Choice

The belief that individuals should be able to make their own choices also shapes attitudes about what abortion policy should be. This powerful impulse is present in many areas of life besides abortion. A Yankelovich Partners question asked in April 1994 found a quarter of respondents agreed with the statement that "smoking is a bad habit and our society should do everything possible to stamp it out." But a huge majority, 73 percent, opted instead for "smoking may be a bad habit, but everyone should have the right to make his or her own choice about whether to smoke or not." Surveys by Gallup for the educational society Phi Delta Kappa have found consistent support for the idea of letting parents choose the schools that their children attend in their local communities; in 1995, 69 percent favored allowing parents to choose. Throughout the debate on President Clinton's health care proposal, people were very skeptical about a health care plan that would limit their individual options.

Questions about pornography reflect the impulse, too. In a February 1996 CBS News/*New York Times* poll, 61 percent of those surveyed said that adults should be permitted to buy or read whatever they wish; only 36 percent said that government at some level should restrict the sale of pornography to adults. An analysis of support for third parties in the fall 1996 issue of *Public Opinion Quarterly* concluded with the observation that "support for a third party seems to be rooted in a desire for more choices at the polls rather than any deep-seated desire to replace, or do away with, the existing choices." Questions about making the abortifacient RU-486 available show that people want to make the choice about using it for themselves. Surveys that probe whether we should allow individuals with terminal illnesses to end their own lives show that we want individual decision making respected.

Survey after survey that discusses abortion in the context of choice reveals broad and deep support for the idea. A poll from the Family Research Council in September 1993 found that 67 percent agreed with the statement "Women should have the right to choose to have an abortion." Other polls that use this formulation find considerable support for allowing a woman to make this choice on her own. For the past nine years, NBC News and the *Wall Street Journal* have asked a question that pulls people in the direction of supporting choice. In each case a majority has said that its opinion is best represented by the statement "The choice on abortion should be left up to the woman and her doctor" (table 5). Another question posed by the same news organizations emphasizes government interference with individual choice; large majorities in 1993 and 1994 agreed that the government should not interfere with a woman's ability to have an abortion (table 6). A more recent question asked in January 1998 by CBS News and the *New York Times* gets at this issue in another way, by asking whether government should stay out of it: "Regardless of your opinion about abortion, do you think the federal government should decide whether abortion should be legal or not, or should each state government decide, or is abortion something the government should stay out of?" Fifty-nine percent said government should stay out of it, 23 percent wanted the federal government to decide, and 14 percent wanted state governments to decide.

Seven times since 1978, Roper Starch Worldwide has asked a question about abortion that highlights individual choice. Respondents were asked whether they were more in favor of or more opposed to a number of different things. When asked about "legal abortions for those women who choose to have them," those surveyed said they were more in favor than more opposed (table 7).

A question asked over the past nineteen years by CBS News/*New York Times* pollsters and by ICR Survey Research confirms this picture. Around six in ten say a woman should be allowed to have an abortion if she wants one and if her doctor agrees (table 8).

Several pollsters ask whether people consider themselves pro-choice or pro-life. Perhaps because of the reach of American individualism, more people describe themselves as pro-choice than pro-life. A Gallup question asked seven times since 1995 found that between 48 and 56 percent considered themselves pro-choice and 34 to 45 percent considered themselves pro-life. In 1998, the responses were 48 percent pro-choice, 45 percent pro-life. In a 1998 Louis Harris and Associates survey, 53 percent said they tended to support pro-choice groups more, and 40 percent said they tended to support pro-life groups more. In the question, the pro-choice groups were described as supporting a woman's right to have an abortion; the pro-life groups were described as opposing abortion.

Abortion Circumstances

As the data above show, Americans place great weight on both the sanctity of life and the importance of individual choice. It follows from this that, in the public mind, women should be able to make their own choices, but their choices should not be unlimited. Thirty-five years ago, Gallup gave us an idea of the limitations people would place on abortion. In 1962, it found support for the idea that abortion should be legal when the health of the mother is in danger (77 percent agreed, 16 percent disagreed) and where the child might be deformed (55 percent agreed, 31 percent disagreed). In both of these cases, the condition of the pregnancy was beyond the woman's control. But also in 1962, only 15 percent said that abortion operations should be legal when "the family does not have enough money to support another child." Seventy-four percent said they should not. Women should be able to have abortions, then, but not because the pregnancy is inconvenient.

In 1972, the National Opinion Research Center (NORC) began asking questions similar to those Gallup wrote in 1962. The *identical* questions have been asked about twenty times in the past twenty-seven years, and they reinforce the point made by the Gallup questions discussed above. By huge majorities, Americans support legal abortion when the woman's own health is seriously endangered by the pregnancy (table 9). Around eight in ten consistently support abortion if there is a strong chance of a serious defect in the baby (table 10). Roughly eight in ten also support legal abortion if the pregnancy is the result of rape (table 11). The responses to these questions have been rock solid for just over a quarter of a century. At the same time, the public is deeply divided about legal abortion if the family has a very low income and cannot afford any more children (table 12), if the woman is married but does not want any more children (table 13), or if she is not married and does not want to marry the man (table 14).

A question that NORC began asking in 1977 finds majorities disagreeing with the concept that a pregnant woman should be able to obtain a legal abortion if she wants one for any reason. In 1998, for example, 56 percent opposed legal abortion in this circumstance; 39 percent supported it. In 1977, 60 percent opposed the availability of legal abortion for any reason, and 37 percent supported it. Taken as a whole, the NORC questions reveal reservations about abortion in situations where a woman can control her fertility. A question asked in 1998 by CBS News and the *New York Times* reinforces this point. Only a quarter of those surveyed said it should be possible for a pregnant woman to obtain a legal abortion if the pregnancy would force a professional woman to interrupt her career. Seven in ten said it should not be possible. As a group, the NORC questions support our belief that abortion opinion is remarkably stable but complex.

Since 1981, ABC News has asked people whether they tended to agree or disagree that "a woman should be able to get an abortion if she decides she wants one no matter what the reason." The results differ from those obtained by NORC. Majorities have usually agreed that this should be possible, though the size of the majorities has varied considerably. In 1998, 50 percent agreed, but 47 percent disagreed (table 15).

In 1991, NORC asked two pairs of questions dealing with legality and also with personal moral judgments about abortion. First, respondents were asked whether the law should or should not allow a pregnant woman to obtain a legal abortion "if there is a strong chance of a serious defect in the baby," and separately, "if the family has a low income and cannot afford any more children." NORC followed up those questions by asking, "Do you personally think it is wrong or not wrong for a woman to have an abortion?" in the circumstance just mentioned. NORC found that 80 percent of the pro-choice group (those supporting legal abortion in both circumstances) thought both that abortion should be legal and that it is not wrong. About a fifth of the pro-choice group, however, were what NORC called "merely tolerant" of abortion, favoring its legality but believing it to be personally wrong.

Because abortion involves what for many people is the taking of life, it is not surprising that the public does not want the procedure undertaken lightly. Large and unvarying majorities support laws requiring doctors to inform patients about alternatives to abortion. Around three-quarters support laws requiring a woman who is seeking an abortion to wait twenty-four hours before having the procedure done.

Seven in ten support spousal notification and parental consent (table 16).

Public support for limitations on abortion can be seen in other areas. In 1975, Harris found 68 percent opposed to legalizing second trimester abortions, and 20 percent wanting them permitted. A question asked by Gallup in August 1996 found nearly two-thirds saying abortion should be generally legal in the first three months, but large majorities saying it should be generally illegal in the second three months (65 percent) and in the final three months (82 percent). Thirteen percent said abortion should be generally legal in the third trimester (table 17). In early 1998, Harris asked a question very similar to Gallup's 1996 question, and the results were virtually identical. Sixty-three percent of those surveyed by Harris said abortion should be legal in the first three months of pregnancy (34 percent disagreed), 26 percent said it should be legal in the second three months (69 percent disagreed), and 13 percent said it should be legal in the third trimester (81 percent disagreed).

In 1998, when CBS News and the *New York Times* asked whether abortion should be "permitted" or "forbidden" in the first three months of pregnancy, 61 percent said it should be permitted, 9 percent volunteered that it depends, 2 percent were not sure, and 28 percent said it should be forbidden. The pollsters then asked those who said it should be permitted, that it depended, or that they weren't sure, whether abortion should be permitted during the second trimester. Fifteen percent said it should be permitted, 16 percent that it depended, and 3 percent were not sure. Thirty-eight percent said it should be forbidden. The pollsters followed this up by asking the remaining supporters and ambivalent respondents whether it should be permitted in the third trimester. Seven percent said it should be permitted, 11 percent volunteered it depended, and 2 percent were not sure. Fourteen percent wanted it forbidden. Although most Americans did not closely follow the recent congressional debates on partial-birth abortions, polls showed that majorities opposed this abortion procedure. The same CBS News/*New York Times* poll, for example, showed that of those who had heard or read about the debate, 73 percent thought it should be outlawed, and 12 percent legal. Of those who thought it should be illegal, 60 percent said it should be legal if the abortion "was necessary to prevent a serious threat to a woman's health."

Abortion Policy

Given this configuration of opinion, what do Americans want abortion policy to be? The data we have compiled for table 18 make clear that Americans do not want to ban abortion. In most polls, six in ten or more oppose a constitutional amendment to outlaw it. Nor do the surveys suggest that Americans want abortion to be legal in all cases. Pluralities or majorities want abortion to be legal only under certain circumstances.

Gallup has one of the longest continuous trends on abortion policy. In 1975, roughly the same percentages of those surveyed said abortion should be legal under any circumstances as said it should be illegal in all circumstances—21 and 22 percent, respectively. A majority, 54 percent, planted themselves firmly in the middle. They wanted abortion legal only under certain circumstances. Twenty-three years later, 59 percent placed themselves in the center. Just under a quarter answered that abortion should be legal under any circumstances, and 17 percent said it should be illegal in all circumstances (table 19).

The University of Michigan's National Election Study (NES) conducts large-scale surveys in election years. The NES asked the same question about abortion in 1972, 1976, 1978, and 1980. In 1980, another abortion question was included, and the new question has been used ever since. The responses to both the old and the new questions are steady. For the question asked between 1972 and 1980, people were given four response categories. In each iteration, only about

11

one in ten said abortion should never be permitted, and around a quarter felt it should never be forbidden, "since one should not require a woman to have a child she doesn't want." Only small numbers say that abortion should be legal for a woman who would have difficulty caring for the child. Pluralities would permit abortion if the life and health of the woman are in danger (table 20). The new question stresses choice and finds between 35 and 46 percent choosing the response "By law, a woman should always be able to obtain an abortion as a matter of personal choice." Almost as many choose the response, "The law should permit abortion only in cases of rape, incest, or when the woman's life is in danger." In this question, once again, roughly one in ten say abortion should never be permitted. A new response category (supported by between 14 and 19 percent over the period 1980 to 1996) states that abortion should be permitted for reasons other than rape or incest or danger to the woman's life, but only after the need has been clearly established (table 21).

A question asked frequently since 1987 by Yankelovich Partners finds that small numbers of people want to outlaw abortion. Majorities or pluralities usually choose the response of making abortion legal in certain circumstances, such as danger to the mother's health, rape, or incest. In the many iterations of this question, between 34 and 49 percent have chosen an option that includes the element of personal choice: "A woman should be able to get an abortion if she decides she wants one, no matter what the reason." In January 1998, 38 percent chose that response (table 22).

In September 1989, CBS News and the *New York Times* began asking a question about abortion that the news organizations have repeated frequently. In 1995, they introduced a new question but continued to repeat the old one. The first question provides three options. Roughly four in ten think it should be available under stricter limits than now. About two in ten say that abortion should not be permitted under any circumstances. Between 32 and 43 percent have

12

said it should be generally available to those who want it (table 23). The new question provides four possible responses. In 1998, a quarter thought it should be generally available and, separately, that it should be available but under stricter limits. Four in ten said it should be against the law except in cases of rape, incest, and to save the mother's life. Nine percent said it should not be permitted at all (table 24).

Louis Harris and Associates has asked on six occasions since 1985 whether abortion should be legal in all, some, or no circumstances, and the results have been generally consistent. In 1998, a majority (58 percent) chose the response that abortion should be legal in some circumstances, about a quarter in all circumstances, and 17 percent in no circumstances (table 25). The final question in this series is also one posed by Harris. A number of survey researchers have reservations about this question because it seems to suggest that *Roe v. Wade* dealt only with the first trimester of pregnancy. This is not the case (see footnote 1 for a discussion of this point). We include the results of this flawed question because it has been asked over a long period (table 26).

Group Responses

Thus far, we have examined attitudes at the national level about abortion. We turn now to the views of different groups in the population. To do this, we use data from the national exit polls conducted by Voter Research and Surveys in 1992 and by Voter News Service and, separately, by the *Los Angeles Times* in 1996.[2] The exit poll samples are large, and they allow us to look with confidence at relatively narrow slices of the population.

2. The 1992 Voter Research and Surveys exit poll consortium was made up of CBS News, NBC News, ABC News, CNN, and the Associated Press. In 1996, Fox News was added to this group and the exit poll consortium became the Voter News Service. The *Los Angeles Times* conducted a separate exit poll in 1996.

In 1992 and 1996, Voter Research and Surveys and its successor, Voter News Service, asked identical questions about abortion. In 1992, 34 percent of voters leaving the polls answered a question on the exit poll "ballot," indicating that "abortion should be legal in all cases" was the statement that came closest to their position. Thirty percent said abortion should be "legal in most cases." About a quarter, 23 percent, said abortion should be illegal in most cases, and 9 percent would make it always illegal. Although nearly four times as many voters said abortion should be always legal as said it should be always illegal, the majority of voters put themselves in the middle categories. The results in 1996 were 25, 35, 24, and 12 percent, respectively (table 27).

Gender differences in voting have become a permanent feature of our politics. In recent elections, men have been more Republican, and women more Democratic. But the abortion issue does not appear to be driving these new allegiances. Men and women do not differ significantly on it. In 1992, slightly more women than men (37 to 31 percent) told the exit pollsters that abortion should be legal in all cases. And slightly more women than men wanted to make it illegal in all cases (10 to 8 percent). In 1996, the pattern was the same. Once again, most men and women planted themselves in one of the two categories in the middle. A person's marital status produces stronger differences on abortion questions than does a person's gender. Married voters are generally older and more Republican than single voters. They are much less accepting of the idea that abortion should be legal in all cases than are single voters, as the table shows.

Age and education are powerful determinants of attitudes on abortion, but even in these areas, it is not possible to find a majority in any age or educational group who wants to make abortion legal in all cases. Nor is it possible to find even two in ten who want to make it illegal in all cases. As the table shows, younger voters are more permissive about abortion policy than are older ones. Voters with higher levels of formal education are more accepting of legal abortion in all cases than are voters with less formal education.

Republicans are less supportive of the idea of making abortion legal in all cases than are Democrats or Independents, but even among Democrats, just 40 percent in 1992 and 33 percent in 1996 said they wanted abortion to be legal in all cases.

Some national surveys have shown that blacks, and particularly black women, are more conservative about abortion than are whites. The exit poll data from 1992 do not show significant differences between black and white voters on this issue; the differences are greater in 1996. In this survey of voters as in other national surveys of adults, Protestants and Catholics look very much alike in their views about abortion. It is Jews and those who profess no religious affiliation who stand apart. A majority of Jews and significant numbers of those with no religious affiliation believe abortion should be legal in all cases.

We include data from the 1996 *Los Angeles Times* exit poll to illustrate a significant new group dynamic in our politics. The religious affiliation of voters is politically consequential, but so, too, is what the psephologists today call their "religiosity." Religiosity means the degree of religious commitment or involvement, and it is explored in the 1996 *Los Angeles Times* exit poll question by asking about the voters' frequency of religious attendance. In table 28, we look at voters' views on abortion by religious denomination and religiosity. As in the exit poll data shown in table 27, Catholics and Protestants look very similar in their views about abortion. Jews and those with no religious affiliation are more likely than Catholics and Protestants to believe abortion ought not to be made illegal. But when we look at religious attendance, we find that Catholics and Protestants who attend religious services regularly look very different on the abortion issue from Catholics and Protestants who attend church rarely. Sixty-two percent of Protestants and 62 percent of Catholics who attend church rarely want abortion not to be illegal. Only 34 percent of Protestants and 27 percent of Catholics who attend church regularly take this view.

Abortion and Elections

If presidential contests are a guide, the abortion issue will continue to get significant election-year attention from the pollsters. In 1996, the pollsters examined abortion attitudes during the primaries, the conventions, and the general election campaign. As we have seen above, they also probed attitudes by asking voters about abortion on Election Day.

During the 1996 campaign, several survey organizations asked people how important the abortion issue would be to them on Election Day. A Louis Harris and Associates poll taken in August 1996 found more than six in ten (62 percent) of those surveyed saying that their votes would not be influenced by the candidates' positions on abortion. Eighteen percent said their votes would be influenced a great deal by this, and 15 percent, quite a lot. Wirthlin Worldwide approached the issue of the importance of abortion differently. In 1992 and again in 1996, the organization asked respondents whether there was any one issue that they felt so strongly about that they would vote for or against a candidate based on that issue alone. In July 1992, 55 percent said there was no such issue. A virtually identical 53 percent gave that response in May 1996. To those who mentioned abortion, Wirthlin Worldwide posed a follow-up question, asking them whether they would vote for a candidate who took a pro-life or a pro-choice position. The results in both years were similar. In 1996, 9 percent said they would vote only for someone who was pro-life, and 6 percent said they would vote only for someone who was pro-choice.

Results of a Gallup question asked in 1992 and again in 1996 are also included in this table. In both years, around three in ten voters said abortion would not be a major issue in their vote for major offices, a plurality said a candidate's position on abortion would be just one of many important factors when voting, and fewer than two in ten said they would vote only for a candidate who shared their views on abortion (table 29). In January 1998, CBS News and the *New*

York Times asked people how much their vote in the next congressional election would be influenced by a candidate's position on abortion. Seven percent said it was the "most important single issue" to them, 57 percent said that "it is important, but so are other issues," and 34 percent said "it won't influence my vote." Ten percent of Republicans, 6 percent of Democrats, and 5 percent of independents indicated it would be the most important issue for them. These surveys and many from previous election years strongly suggest that abortion is not a pivotal issue for the vast majority of voters.

As it has in past election years, the abortion issue received substantial media coverage during the political conventions of 1996. Given their level of interest and activism in politics, convention delegates and party activists often have views on issues that are stronger or purer than those of the public. As polls of convention delegates on a wide variety of issues show, Democratic delegates are generally more liberal than members of their own party and the population, and Republican delegates are more conservative than other Republicans and the population. This pattern holds true on abortion, and the data in table 30 illustrate the point. Sixty-one percent of Democratic delegates told CBS News/*New York Times* pollsters that they personally felt abortion should be permitted in all cases. Thirty percent of self-identified Democrats felt that way, as did about 27 percent of registered voters. Twenty-one percent of self-identified Republicans agreed as did only 11 percent of delegates to the Republican convention. As table 31 shows, majorities of delegates to the 1988, 1992, and 1996 GOP and Democratic conventions disagreed with the view that there should be a constitutional amendment outlawing abortion, but the Democratic delegates are much more adamant about this than are the Republican delegates.

In most of the exit polls, pollsters have included a simple question asking voters to select from a list the one or two issues that had the most effect on their vote. The questions have been worded slightly differently, and in some presidential years, abortion has not been included in the list of issues people could check off on their "ballots." In 1996, the *Los Angeles Times* exit poll included abortion in its list of possible responses to the question: "Which issues—if any—were most important to you in deciding how you would vote for president today?" Voters were told to choose up to two responses. Forty percent checked moral and ethical values, and 35 percent, jobs and the economy. Nine percent of voters said abortion was most important to them. Six percent of Clinton voters, 13 percent of those who voted for Dole, and 5 percent of those who chose Perot selected abortion as most important to them. Of the 9 percent of all voters who selected abortion, 60 percent voted for Dole and 34 percent for Clinton (table 32).

As table 32 shows, the results from exit polls in earlier presidential contests are roughly consistent with the *Los Angeles Times* results. Small numbers of voters have said that abortion was the most important issue to them in casting their votes, and at this level, the issue has been a plus for the GOP. As single-issue votes go, these small numbers are not insignificant. The group of voters is larger than the number who mention "the environment," for example, but smaller than the number who usually say economic issues are central to their voting decision.[3]

Opinion on abortion remains very much what it was in 1973 when the *Roe v. Wade* decision was handed down. Americans do not want to outlaw abortion, but neither do they think it should be completely unrestricted. Their views are at once complex and clear.

———————

3. See *Attitudes toward the Environment: Twenty-five Years after Earth Day*, Everett Carll Ladd and Karlyn H. Bowman (Washington, D.C.: AEI Press, 1995), p. 46.

TABLE 1
ABORTION AS MURDER, 1983–1998
(percent)

QUESTION: Which of these statements comes closer to your opinion—abortion is the same thing as murdering a child, OR abortion is not murder because a fetus isn't a person? (1983–1987)

QUESTION: Which of these statements comes closer to your opinion: abortion is the same thing as murdering a child, OR abortion is not murder because the fetus really isn't a child? (1989–1998)

	Murder	Not Murder	Depends[a]
Nov. 1983[b]	57	30	na
Nov. 1985	54	35	na
Dec. 1985	55	35	na
Aug. 1987	50	35	na
Apr. 1989	48	40	4
July 1989[c]	40	47	7
Jan. 1995	46	41	5
Jan. 1998	50	38	5

na = not available.

a. Volunteered responses.

b. *New York Times* only.

c. Question read ". . . abortion is not murder because the fetus really hasn't developed into a child yet."

SOURCE: Surveys by CBS News/*New York Times*, latest that of January 1998.

TABLE 2
ABORTION AS MURDER, 1994–1998
(percent)

QUESTION: Some people say that abortion is an act of murder, while other people disagree with this. What is your view—do you think that abortion is an act of murder or don't you feel this way?

	An Act of Murder	Don't Feel This Way
Aug. 1994	43	47
Jan. 1995	40	51
Jan. 1998	48	45

SOURCE: Surveys by Yankelovich Partners for *Time*/CNN (1994–1995) and the Gallup Organization (1998), latest that of January 1998.

TABLE 3
PERSONAL VIEWS ABOUT ABORTION, 1996
(percent)

QUESTION: Would you say you are personally for or against abortion?

	For	Against	Not Sure[a]
May 1996	38	44	18
Aug. 1996	34	48	17

a. Volunteered responses.
SOURCE: Surveys by Opinion Dynamics for Fox News, latest that of August 1996.

TABLE 4
ABORTION—GOOD AND BAD EFFECTS, 1992 AND 1995
(percent)

QUESTION: Many things in our society have both good and bad effects. For example, aviation does because it provides fast transportation. Here is a list of some different things that have resulted in both good and bad effects. [Card is shown to respondent.] Would you read down the list and for each one tell me whether, on balance, you think the good effects outweigh the bad, or whether the bad effects outweigh the good? . . . Abortion.

	Good Outweighs Bad	Bad Outweighs Good	Equally Good and Bad[a]
Mar. 1992	24	47	20
Mar. 1995	24	47	21

a. Volunteered responses.
SOURCE: Surveys by Roper Starch Worldwide, latest that of March 1995.

TABLE 5
A WOMAN'S CHOICE? 1990–1998
(percent)

QUESTION: Which of the following best represents your views about abortion? (1) The choice on abortion should be left up to the woman and her doctor; (2) Abortion should be legal only in cases where pregnancy results from rape or incest, or when the life of the woman is at risk; (3) Abortion should be illegal in all circumstances.

	Choice between a Woman and Her Doctor	Legal Only in Cases of Rape and Incest or When Mother's Life Is at Risk	Illegal in All Circumstances
July 1990	57	33	8
June 1991	57	36	7
July 1991	60	31	8
Dec. 1995	60	28	10
Mar. 1996	56	31	10
May 1996	55	35	7
June 1996	58	31	9
Aug. 1996	56	30	12
Sept. 1996	58	30	9
Jan. 1998	60	26	11

SOURCE: Surveys by Hart/Teeter Research for NBC News/*Wall Street Journal,* latest that of January 1998.

TABLE 6
GOVERNMENT INTERFERENCE, 1993–1994
(percent)

QUESTION: I would like to read several statements about some social issues facing America. For each issue, please tell me whether you agree strongly, agree somewhat, disagree somewhat, or disagree strongly with that statement. . . : The government should not interfere with a woman's ability to have an abortion.

	Agree Strongly	Agree Somewhat	Disagree Somewhat	Disagree Strongly
June 1993[a]	63	12	7	14
June 1994	53	17	9	18

a. Question wording read, ". . . woman's right to have an abortion."

SOURCE: Surveys by Hart/Teeter Research for NBC News/*Wall Street Journal*, latest that of June 1994.

TABLE 7
LEGAL ABORTIONS FOR WOMEN WHO CHOOSE TO HAVE THEM, 1978–1998
(percent)

QUESTION: Frequently on any controversial issue there is no clear-cut side that people take, and also frequently solutions on controversial issues are worked out by compromise. But I'm going to name some different things, and for each one would you tell me whether on balance you would be more in favor of it, or more opposed to it? . . . Legal abortions for those women who choose to have them.

	Favor	Oppose	Mixed Feelings/Don't Know
1978	46	42	12
1981	46	42	12
1984	47	39	15
1989	46	38	16
1993	49	36	15
1995	49	35	16
1998	48	37	15

SOURCE: Surveys by Roper Starch Worldwide, latest that of October 1998.

TABLE 8
SHOULD A WOMAN BE ALLOWED TO
HAVE AN ABORTION? 1980–1998
(percent)

QUESTION: If a woman wants to have an abortion, and her doctor agrees to it, should she be allowed to have an abortion, or not?

	Should	Should Not	Depends[a]
Aug. 1980	62	19	15
Apr. 1981	63	25	9
June 1981	65	22	10
Jan. 1989	61	25	11
Apr. 1989	63	24	10
July 1989	63	24	11
Sept. 1989	58	26	13
June 1992	58	20	16
Feb. 1995	66	22	11
Jan. 1998	59	24	14

a. Volunteered responses.
SOURCE: Surveys by CBS News/*New York Times* (1980–1989, 1998) and ICR Survey Research for Associated Press (1992–1995), latest that of January 1998.

TABLE 9
ABORTION IF A WOMAN'S HEALTH IS IN
SERIOUS DANGER? 1972–1998
(percent)

QUESTION: Please tell me whether or not you think it should be possible for a pregnant woman to obtain a legal abortion if a woman's own health is seriously endangered by the pregnancy?

	Yes	*No*
1972	83	13
1973	91	8
1974	90	7
1975	88	9
1976	89	9
1977	89	9
1978	88	9
1980	88	10
1982	90	8
1983	87	10
1984	88	10
1985	87	10
1987	86	11
1988	86	11
1989	88	10
1990	89	8
1993	86	10
1994	88	9
1996	89	8
1998	88	7
1998	84	12

SOURCE: Surveys by National Opinion Research Center (1972–1996, second 1998) and CBS News/*New York Times* (first 1998), latest that of 1998.

TABLE 10
ABORTION IF THERE IS A CHANCE OF
SERIOUS DEFECT IN BABY? 1972–1998
(percent)

QUESTION: Please tell me whether or not you think it should be possible for a pregnant woman to obtain a legal abortion if there is a strong chance of a serious defect in the baby?

	Yes	No
1972	75	20
1973	82	15
1974	83	14
1975	80	16
1976	82	16
1977	83	14
1978	80	18
1980	80	16
1982	81	15
1983	76	20
1984	78	19
1985	76	21
1987	77	20
1988	76	21
1989	79	18
1990	78	18
1991	80	16
1993	79	18
1994	80	17
1996	79	18
1998	75	18
1998	75	21

SOURCE: Surveys by National Opinion Research Center (1972–1996, second 1998) and CBS News/*New York Times* (first 1998), latest that of 1998.

TABLE 11
ABORTION IF THE PREGNANCY IS A RESULT OF RAPE? 1972–1998
(percent)

QUESTION: Please tell me whether or not you think it should be possible for a pregnant woman to obtain a legal abortion if she became pregnant as a result of rape?

	Yes	No
1972	75	20
1973	81	16
1974	83	13
1975	80	16
1976	81	16
1977	81	16
1978	81	16
1980	80	16
1982	83	13
1983	80	16
1984	77	19
1985	78	18
1987	78	18
1988	77	18
1989	80	16
1990	81	15
1991	83	13
1993	79	16
1994	81	16
1996	81	15
1998	84	12
1998	77	19

SOURCE: Surveys by National Opinion Research Center (1972–1996, second 1998) and CBS News/*New York Times* (first 1998), latest that of 1998.

TABLE 12
ABORTION IF A FAMILY HAS VERY LOW INCOME AND CANNOT
AFFORD ANY MORE CHILDREN? 1972–1998
(percent)

QUESTION: Please tell me whether or not you think it should be possible for a pregnant woman to obtain a legal abortion if the family has a very low income and cannot afford any more children?

	Yes	No
1972	46	48
1973	52	45
1974	52	43
1975	51	45
1976	51	45
1977	52	45
1978	46	51
1980	50	46
1982	50	46
1983	42	54
1984	45	52
1985	42	55
1987	44	53
1988	41	56
1989	46	50
1990	46	49
1991	47	49
1993	48	48
1994	49	48
1996	45	51
1998	43	54
1998	42	53

SOURCE: Surveys by National Opinion Research Center (1972–1996, second 1998) and CBS News/*New York Times* (first 1998), latest that of 1998.

TABLE 13
ABORTION IF A WOMAN IS MARRIED AND
DOES NOT WANT MORE CHILDREN? 1972–1998
(percent)

QUESTION: Please tell me whether or not you think it should be possible for a pregnant woman to obtain a legal abortion if she is married and does not want any more children?

	Yes	No
1972	38	57
1973	46	51
1974	45	50
1975	44	52
1976	45	52
1977	45	51
1978	39	58
1980	45	51
1982	46	49
1983	38	59
1984	41	56
1985	39	58
1987	40	56
1988	39	58
1989	43	54
1990	43	53
1991	43	53
1993	45	50
1994	47	50
1996	45	51
1998	39	55
1998	40	55

SOURCE: Surveys by National Opinion Research Center (1972–1996, second 1998) and CBS News/*New York Times* (first 1998), latest that of 1998.

TABLE 14
ABORTION IF A WOMAN IS NOT MARRIED AND DOES NOT WANT TO MARRY THE MAN? 1972–1998
(percent)

QUESTION: Please tell me whether or not you think it should be possible for a pregnant woman to obtain a legal abortion if she is not married and does not want to marry the man?

	Yes	No
1972	41	53
1973	47	49
1974	48	48
1975	46	49
1976	48	48
1977	48	48
1978	40	57
1980	46	49
1982	47	49
1983	38	58
1984	43	54
1985	40	57
1987	40	56
1988	38	58
1989	43	52
1990	43	52
1991	43	53
1993	46	49
1994	46	51
1996	43	53
1998	35	62
1998	40	55

SOURCE: Surveys by National Opinion Research Center (1972–1996, second 1998) and CBS News/*New York Times* (first 1998), latest that of 1998.

TABLE 15
ABORTION FOR ANY REASON? 1977–1998
(percent)

QUESTION: Please tell me whether or not you think it should be possible for a pregnant woman to obtain a legal abortion if she wants one for any reason? (NORC)

	Yes	No
1977	37	60
1978	32	65
1980	39	57
1982	39	56
1983	33	64
1984	37	60
1985	36	61
1987	38	58
1988	35	61
1989	39	57
1990	42	54
1991	41	51
1993	43	52
1994	45	52
1996	43	52
1998	39	56

QUESTION: On another subject, do you tend to agree or disagree with this statement: A woman should be able to get an abortion if she decides she wants one no matter what the reason? (ABC/WP)

	Agree	Disagree
May 1981	40	59
Jan. 1985	52	46
Feb. 1986	54	44
Aug. 1987	53	44
Feb. 1989	50	49
Oct. 1989	54	45
July 1990	54	46
June 1991	57	41
Aug. 1993	59	40
Aug. 1994	64	34
Jan. 1998	50	47

SOURCE: Surveys by National Opinion Research Center and ABC News/*Washington Post*, latest that of 1998.

TABLE 16
VIEWS ON LAWS LIMITING ABORTION, 1989–1998
(percent)

QUESTION: Do you favor or oppose each of the following proposals. . . ?

	Favor	Oppose
A law requiring women seeking abortions to wait 24 hours before having the procedure done		
Jan. 1992	73	23
July 1996	74	22
Jan. 1998[a]	79	16
A law requiring doctors to inform patients about alternatives to abortion before performing procedure		
Jan. 1992	86	12
July 1996	86	11
A law requiring women under 18 to get parental consent for any abortion		
July 1989[a]	60	28
Jan. 1992	70	23
July 1996	74	23
Jan. 1998[a]	78	17
A law requiring that the husband of a married woman be notified if she decides to have an abortion		
Jan. 1992	73	25
July 1996	70	26

a. Question wording varied slightly.
SOURCE: Surveys by CBS News/*New York Times* (1989, 1998) and the Gallup Organization for CNN/*USA Today* (1992, 1996), latest that of January 1998.

TABLE 17
Stages of Pregnancy and the Question of Legality, 1996
(percent)

QUESTION: Thinking more generally, do you think abortion should be generally legal or generally illegal during each of the following stages of pregnancy?

	Should Be Generally Legal	Should Be Generally Illegal	Depends[a]
In the first three months of pregnancy	64	30	4
In the second three months of pregnancy	26	65	7
In the last three months of pregnancy	13	82	3

NOTE: A Field (California) poll taken in February 1997 found that 62 percent of Californians approve of allowing abortions in the first three months of pregnancy; 26 percent approved of allowing them in the second three months, and 14 percent approved of allowing the procedure in the last trimester of pregnancy.

a. Volunteered responses.

SOURCE: Survey by the Gallup Organization for CNN/USA Today, August 1996.

TABLE 18
Constitutional Amendment to Ban Abortion, 1982–1998
(percent)

QUESTION: Do you favor or oppose . . . a constitutional amendment to ban legalized abortion?

	Organization	Favor	Oppose
Feb. 1982	Harris	33	61
July 1982	Harris	31	62
Mar. 1984	Harris	33	62
July 1987	Harris	33	62
Jan. 1989	Harris	29	68

QUESTION: Do you favor or oppose . . . a constitutional amendment to ban abortions?

	Organization	Favor	Oppose
Apr. 1984	Harris	34	59
Sept. 1984	Harris	31	63
Sept. 1984	Harris	20	61
Jan. 1985	Harris	38	58
Sept. 1985	Harris	37	55

QUESTION: Do you favor or oppose each of the following . . . a constitutional amendment to ban all abortions?

	Organization	Favor	Oppose
Feb. 1996	Yankelovich	24	70
Mar. 1996	Yankelovich	21	70
May 1996	Yankelovich	28	64

QUESTION: Would you favor or oppose an amendment to the Constitution which would make all abortions illegal?

	Organization	Favor	Oppose
Sept. 1982	CBS/*NYT*	28	68
Jan. 1998	CBS/*NYT*	22	76

SOURCE: Surveys by Louis Harris and Associates, Inc., Yankelovich Partners for *Time*/CNN and CBS News/*New York Times*, latest that of January 1998.

TABLE 19
CIRCUMSTANCES UNDER WHICH ABORTION SHOULD BE LEGAL, 1975–1998
(percent)

QUESTION: Do you think abortions should be legal under any circumstances, legal only under certain circumstances, or illegal in all circumstances?

	Legal under Any Circumstances	Legal Only under Certain Circumstances	Illegal in All Circumstances
1975	21	54	22
1977	22	55	19
1979	22	54	19
1980	25	53	18
1981	23	52	21
1983	23	58	16
1988	24	57	17
Apr. 1989	27	50	18
July 1989	29	51	17
Apr. 1990	31	53	12
May 1991	32	50	17
Sept. 1991	33	49	14
Jan. 1992	31	53	14
June 1992	34	48	13
Mar. 1993	32	51	13

Mar. 1994	31	51	15
Sept. 1994	33	52	13
Feb. 1995	33	50	15
Sept. 1995	31	54	12
July 1996	25	58	15
Sept. 1996	23	51	18
Aug. 1997	22	61	15
Nov. 1997	26	55	17
Jan. 1998	23	59	17

	Most Circumstances	Only a Few Circumstances
Sept. 1994	13	37
Feb. 1995	9	41
Sept. 1995	14	39
July 1996	13	43
Sept. 1996	13	37
Aug. 1997	12	48
Nov. 1997	15	40
Jan. 1998	16	42

NOTE: Since September 1994, those who said, "Abortion should be legal only under certain circumstances," were asked this follow-up question: "Do you think abortion should be legal under most circumstances or only in a few circumstances?"

SOURCE: Surveys by the Gallup Organization for CNN/*USA Today*, latest that of January 1998.

TABLE 20
WHEN ABORTION SHOULD BE PERMITTED, PART ONE, 1972–1980
(percent)

QUESTION: There has been some discussion about abortion during recent years. Which one of the opinions on this page best agrees with your view? (1) Abortion should never be permitted, (2) Abortion should be permitted only if the life and health of the woman is in danger; (3) Abortion should be permitted if, due to personal reasons, the woman would have difficulty in caring for the child; or (4) Abortion should never be forbidden, since one should not require a woman to have a child she doesn't want.

	Never Permitted	Only If Life and Health in Danger	Personal Difficulty	Should Never Be Forbidden
1972	11	46	17	24
1976	11	44	16	26
1978	10	43	16	26
1980	10	44	18	27

NOTE: In 1972 and 1976, the question began, "Still on the subject of women's rights. . . ."
SOURCE: Surveys by the University of Michigan for the National Election Studies, latest that of 1980.

TABLE 21
WHEN ABORTION SHOULD BE PERMITTED, PART TWO, 1980–1996
(percent)

QUESTION: There has been some discussion about abortion during recent years. Which one of the opinions on this page best agrees with your view? (1) By law, abortion should never be permitted; (2) The law should permit abortion only in cases of rape, incest, or when the woman's life is in danger; (3) The law should permit abortion for reasons other than rape, incest, or danger to the woman's life, but only after the need for the abortion has been clearly established; or (4) By law, a woman should always be able to obtain an abortion as a matter of personal choice.

	Never Permitted	Only in Cases of Rape, Incest, or Danger	Clear Need	Always as Personal Choice
1980	11	32	18	35
1982	13	30	19	35
1984	13	29	19	35
1986	13	28	18	38
1988	12	33	18	35
1990	12	33	14	40
1992	10	28	14	46
1994	12	30	14	42
1996	12	29	16	42

SOURCE: Surveys by the University of Michigan for the National Election Studies, latest that of 1996.

TABLE 22
ABORTION POSITION THAT BEST REPRESENTS YOUR VIEWS, 1987–1998
(percent)

QUESTION: Which of these positions best represents your views about abortion? (1) A woman should be able to get an abortion if she decides she wants one, no matter what the reason; (2) Abortion should only be legal in certain circumstances, such as when a woman's health is endangered or when the pregnancy results from rape or incest; (3) Abortion should be illegal in all circumstances.

	Woman's Decision No Matter What the Reason	Legal in Certain Circumstances	Illegal in All Circumstances
Aug. 1987	34	51	12
Apr. 1989	37	51	9
July 1989	38	50	9
Apr. 1990	43	45	9
May 1990	43	43	10
July 1991	44	44	11
Apr. 1992	47	37	10
Aug. 1992	49	38	12
Jan. 1993	43	43	10
Aug. 1993	47	37	11
Jan. 1994	45	39	13
May 1994	47	39	12
Sept. 1995	44	43	10
May 1996	40	46	11
Jan. 1998	38	43	16

SOURCE: Surveys by Yankelovich Partners for *Time*/CNN, latest that of January 1998.

TABLE 23
ABORTION POSITION CLOSEST TO YOUR VIEW, 1989–1998
(percent)

QUESTION: Which comes closest to your view? (1) Abortion should be generally available to those who want it; or (2) Abortion should be available but under stricter limits than it is now; or (3) Abortion should not be permitted.

	Generally Available	Stricter Limits	Not Permitted
Sept. 1989[a]	40	40	18
Nov. 1989	41	42	15
Jan. 1990	39	40	18
Aug. 1990	41	41	16
June 1991	37	38	22
Aug. 1991	41	40	15
Sept. 1991	42	38	18
Jan. 1992	40	39	19
Mar. 1992	44	37	17
June 1992	42	39	17
June 1992	43	39	16
July 1992	41	39	18
Aug. 1992	41	40	17
Oct. 1992	43	37	16
Mar. 1993	42	36	20
July 1994	40	37	21
Jan. 1995	40	37	21
Jan. 1995	38	37	23
Feb. 1995	43	38	18
Apr. 1995	38	40	20
Aug. 1995	40	36	22
Oct. 1995	37	41	20
Feb. 1996	40	41	18
Apr. 1996	37	41	21
June 1996	35	41	20
July 1996	37	42	19
Jan. 1998	32	45	22

a. Varied wording: (2) Abortion should be available but more difficult to get than it is now, or (3) Abortion should not be available.
SOURCE: Surveys by CBS News/*New York Times*, latest that of January 1998.

TABLE 24
Position Closest to Your General View, 1995–1998
(percent)

QUESTION: Which of these comes closest to your general view? (1) Abortion should be generally available to those who want it; (2) Abortion should be available but under stricter limits than it is now; (3) Abortion should be against the law except in cases of rape, incest, and to save the woman's life; or (4) Abortion should not be permitted at all.

	Generally Available	Available but under Stricter Limits	Against the Law except for Rape, Incest, Mother's Life	Not Permitted
Apr. 1995	35	20	36	8
Aug. 1995	36	20	34	9
Oct. 1995	35	22	36	6
Feb. 1996	36	22	34	7
Apr. 1996	37	17	34	10
June 1996	36	18	37	8
July 1996	33	21	34	9
Jan. 1998	25	25	41	9

SOURCE: Surveys by CBS News/*New York Times*, latest that of January 1998.

TABLE 25
ABORTION IN WHICH CIRCUMSTANCES? 1985–1998
(percent)

QUESTION: In general, do you favor permitting a woman who wants one to have an abortion in all circumstances, some circumstances, or no circumstances?

	All Circumstances	Some Circumstances	No Circumstances
1985	26	53	20
1992	29	54	14
1992	34	52	11
1993	30	55	14
1996	25	53	19
1998	23	58	17

SOURCE: Surveys by Louis Harris and Associates Inc., latest that of January 1998.

TABLE 26
ATTITUDES TOWARD ABORTIONS UP TO THREE MONTHS, 1972–1998
(percent)

QUESTION: In 1973, the U.S. Supreme Court decided that state laws which made it illegal for a woman to have an abortion up to three months of pregnancy were unconstitutional, and that the decision on whether a woman should have an abortion up to three months of pregnancy should be left to the woman and her doctor to decide. In general, do you favor or oppose this part of the U.S. Supreme Court decision making abortions up to three months of pregnancy legal?

	Favor	Oppose	Not Sure
1972	42	46	12
1973	52	42	7
1976	59	28	13
1979	60	37	3
1981	56	41	3
1985	50	47	3
1989	59	37	4
1991	65	33	2
1992	61	35	4
1993	56	42	3
1996	52	41	7
1998	57	41	2

SOURCE: Surveys by Louis Harris and Associates, Inc., latest that of January 1998.

TABLE 27

VIEWS OF DIFFERENT GROUPS OF VOTERS ABOUT ABORTION, 1992 AND 1996
(percent)

QUESTION: Which comes closest to your position? Abortion should be . . .

| | 1992 | | | 1996 | | |
	Legal, all cases	Legal, most cases	Illegal, most cases	Illegal, all cases	Legal, all cases	Legal, most cases	Illegal, most cases	Illegal, all cases
All voters	34	30	23	9	25	35	24	12
Men	31	32	25	8	22	36	27	11
Women	37	28	22	10	28	33	22	13
Married	30	30	26	10	—	—	—	—
Single	43	29	18	7	—	—	—	—
18–29 years	41	27	21	8	29	35	22	11
Men	37	30	22	9	24	39	27	9
Women	44	24	20	8	33	32	18	14
30–44 years	34	32	23	8	29	33	23	11
Men	29	36	25	6	26	35	26	10
Women	37	28	21	10	32	31	21	13

(table continues)

TABLE 27 (continued)

QUESTION: Which comes closest to your position? Abortion should be . . .

	1992						1996				
	Legal, all cases	Legal, most cases	Illegal, most cases	Illegal, all cases			Legal, all cases	Legal, most cases	Illegal, most cases	Illegal, all cases	
45–59 years											
Men	31	31	26	9			22	36	27	10	
Women	28	32	28	8			19	41	26	10	
	35	30	24	8			26	32	28	11	
60+ years	30	27	24	11			17	35	26	15	
Men	31	26	26	11			17	32	31	15	
Women	30	28	22	12			19	37	20	15	
< High school grad.	26	22	27	15			20	34	26	14	
High school grad.	27	30	26	12			20	35	27	13	
Some college	36	30	23	8			22	37	25	12	
College grad.	35	31	23	7			28	30	24	13	
Postgrad.	43	29	20	6			32	37	20	8	
Democrat	40	31	17	7			33	39	17	8	
Men	38	33	18	6			30	42	16	8	
Women	42	30	16	7			36	35	17	8	

Republican								
Men	25	28	32	12	16	29	33	19
Women	23	31	34	11	14	31	37	16
	28	26	29	13	20	26	28	23
Independent/other								
Men	37	30	22	8	24	38	25	8
Women	34	34	23	6	23	37	28	8
	40	27	22	8	25	38	22	9
White	34	30	24	9	24	34	25	12
Black	38	29	17	9	28	39	18	8
Hispanic	31	26	25	16	26	32	24	12
Asian	22	30	27	13	—	—	—	—
Protestant	30	31	26	9	21	35	28	13
Catholic	30	29	26	10	22	37	25	12
Jewish	62	31	5	1	51	40	5	1
Other Christian	28	25	29	15	19	29	31	18
None	60	32	4	2	46	36	9	5

NOTE: The marital status category was presented differently in 1996, so the data are not comparable. Voter News Service (VNS) did not report the results for Asians in 1996 for this question.

SOURCE: Surveys by Voter Research and Surveys, a consortium of ABC News, Associated Press, CBS News, CNN, and NBC News, November 3, 1992, and by VNS, a consortium of ABC News, Associated Press, CBS News, CNN, Fox News, and NBC News, November 5, 1996.

TABLE 28
ABORTION ATTITUDES BY DENOMINATION
AND PARTICIPATION, 1996
(percent)

QUESTION: Do you think abortion should be made illegal in all cases, except for rape, incest, and to save the life of the mother? [Put an X in the box.] Yes, made illegal with exceptions; Yes, made illegal without any exception; No, not made illegal.

QUESTION: What religion do you consider yourself? [Put an X in the box.] Protestant, Roman Catholic, Other Christian, Jewish, Other religion, No religion.

QUESTION: How frequently do you attend religious services, or do you never attend religious services? [Put an X in the box.] (1) Never; (2) Less than once a year; (3) Once a year; (4) Several times a year; (5) Once a month; (6) Several times a month; (7) Once a week; (8) Several times a week; (9) Once a day; (10) Several times a day.

	Not Illegal	Illegal with Exceptions	Illegal Always
Protestant	48	41	11
Catholic	46	41	14
Other Christian	41	44	15
Jewish	74	21	5
No religion	80	16	5
Attend church rarely[a]			
Protestant	62	33	5
Catholic	62	33	5
Other Christian	59	34	7
Attend church regularly			
Protestant	34	50	17
Catholic	27	50	23
Other Christian	22	55	23

NOTE: *Rarely* is the combination of responses 1–4, *Regularly* is the combination of responses 8–10.

a. This part of the table is to be read in this way: of those Protestants and Catholics who attend church rarely, 62 percent think abortion should not be made illegal.

SOURCE: Survey by the *Los Angeles Times,* November 5, 1996.

TABLE 29
ABORTION AS AN ELECTION ISSUE, 1992 AND 1996
(percent)

QUESTION: Is there any one issue that you feel so strongly about that you would vote for or against a candidate based on that issue alone?

	No One Issue	Abortion— Oppose	Abortion— Favor
July 1992	55	10	8
May 1996	53	9	6

QUESTION: Thinking about how the abortion issue might affect your vote for major offices, would you: Only vote for a candidate who shares your views on abortion; or Consider a candidate's position on abortion as just one of many important factors when voting; or Not see abortion as a major issue?

	Only Vote for Candidate Who Shares Views	Just One of Many Important Factors	Not See Abortion as Major Issue
June 1992	13	46	36
July 1996	18	48	30
July 1996	16	51	30
Men	13	51	33
Women	19	51	27

SOURCE: For upper panel, surveys by Wirthlin Worldwide, latest that of May 1996. For lower panel, surveys by the Gallup Organization, latest that of July 1996.

TABLE 30
CONVENTION DELEGATES, PARTISANS, AND VOTERS, 1996
(percent)

QUESTION: What is your personal feeling about abortion:
(1) It should be permitted in all cases; (2) It should be
permitted, but subject to greater restrictions than it is now;
(3) It should be permitted in such cases as rape, incest, and
to save the woman's life; or (4) It should only be permitted
to save the woman's life?

	Permitted in all Cases	Permitted with Some Restrictions	Permitted for Rape/ Incest/ Life	Only to Save Life	Not Permitted at All[a]
Dem. del.[b]	61	15	13	3	—
Dem.[c]	30	11	41	13	2
R.V.[d]	27	14	39	14	3
Rep.[e]	21	16	39	18	4
Rep. del.[f]	11	12	38	27	4

QUESTION: Do you think making abortion illegal is the kind
of issue you would like to change the Constitution for, or
isn't abortion that kind of issue?

	Kind of Issue	Not That Kind of Issue
Dem. del.[b]	3	96
Dem.[c]	22	71
R.V.[d]	22	71
Rep.[e]	24	69
Rep. del.[f]	34	57

NOTE: All categories shown here excepting the delegates were in-
terviewed in August 1996.
a. Volunteered responses.
b. Democratic delegates.
c. Democrats.
d. Registered voters.
e. Republicans.
f. Republican delegates.
SOURCE: Surveys by CBS News/New York Times, 1996.

TABLE 31
CONSTITUTIONAL AMENDMENT ON ABORTION?
THE PUBLIC AND CONVENTION DELEGATES, 1988–1996
(percent)

QUESTION: Do you agree or disagree with the following
statement: There should be a constitutional amendment
outlawing abortion?

	Agree	Disagree
Republican delegates		
1988	36	53
1992	28	55
1996	36	58
General population		
July 1992	25	67
June 1996	24	75
Aug. 1996	26	72
Democratic delegates		
1980	10	na
1984	9	83
1988	6	87
1992	3	93
1996	1	98

na = not available.
SOURCE: Surveys by ABC News/*Washington Post,* latest that of 1996.

TABLE 32
ABORTION AS A VOTING ISSUE ON ELECTION DAY, 1980–1996
(percent)

QUESTION IN 1980: Which issues were most important in deciding how you voted today?[a]

ERA/Abortion Most Important	Voted for Reagan	Voted for Carter
7	38	50

QUESTION IN 1984: Which issues mattered most in deciding how you voted?[b]

Abortion One of Most Important Issues	Voted for Reagan	Voted for Mondale
8	71	28

QUESTION IN 1988: Were any of the items [listed on survey ballot] very important in making your presidential choice?[c]

Abortion Was Very Important	Voted for Bush	Voted for Dukakis
33	54	45

QUESTION IN 1988: Which issues mattered most in deciding how you voted today?[d]

Abortion One of Most Important Issues	Voted for Bush	Voted for Dukakis
7	65	33

QUESTION IN 1988: Which issues—if any—were most important to you in deciding how you would vote today?[e]

Abortion Was Most Important Issue	Voted for Bush	Voted for Dukakis
20	63	36

(*table continues*)

TABLE 32 (continued)

QUESTION IN 1992: Which one or two issues mattered most in deciding how you voted?[d]

Abortion Was an Issue That Mattered Most	Voted for Bush	Voted for Clinton	Voted for Perot
12	55	36	9

QUESTION IN 1996: Which issues—if any—were most important to you in deciding how you would vote for president today?[f]

Abortion Was Most Important	Voted for Dole	Voted for Clinton	Voted for Perot
9	60	34	4

a. Voters could choose up to two responses from a list of eight. "ERA/abortion" was a single category.
b. Voters could choose up to two responses from a list of eight, including "none of these."
c. "The candidates' stand on abortion" was one of twenty-one items listed, including "none of the above."
d. Voters could choose up to two responses from a list of nine.
e. Voters could choose up to two responses from a list of eleven, including "none."
f. Voters could choose up to two responses from a list of eleven, including "none of the above."
SOURCES: For 1980, 1984, and second 1988 question, survey by the *CBS News/New York Times* Exit Poll; for first 1988 question, survey by ABC News Exit Poll; for third 1988 question and 1996, survey by the *Los Angeles Times* Exit Poll; and for 1992, survey by Voter Research and Surveys Exit Poll.

About the Authors

EVERETT CARLL LADD is the director of the Institute for Social Inquiry at the University of Connecticut. He is also the executive director and president of the Roper Center for Public Opinion Research, a private, nonprofit research facility affiliated with the University of Connecticut since 1977.

Mr. Ladd's principal research interests are American political thought, public opinion, and political parties. Among his ten books are *American Political Parties: Ideology in America; Transformations of the American Party System; Where Have All the Voters Gone?* and *The American Polity* (all published by W. W. Norton).

An AEI adjunct scholar, he is a contributor to *Intellectual Capital.com* and to the *Weekly Standard,* a member of the editorial boards of four magazines, and the editor of the Roper Center's magazine, *Public Perspective.* He has been a fellow of the Ford, Guggenheim, and Rockefeller Foundations; the Center for International Studies at Harvard; the Hoover Institution at Stanford; and the Center for Advanced Study in the Behavioral Sciences.

KARLYN H. BOWMAN is a resident fellow at the American Enterprise Institute. She joined AEI in 1979, and was managing editor of *Public Opinion* until 1990. From 1990 to 1995 she was the editor of *The American Enterprise.* Ms. Bowman continues as editor of the magazine's "Opinion Pulse" section, and she writes about public opinion and demographics. Her most recent publications include *What's Wrong: A Survey of American Satisfaction and Complaint* (with Everett Carll Ladd, AEI Press, 1998); *Attitudes toward Economic Inequality* (with Ladd, AEI Press, 1998); *Public Opinion in America and Japan* (with Ladd, AEI Press, 1996); and *The 1993–1994 Debate on Health Care Reform: Did the Polls Mislead the Policy Makers?* (AEI Press, 1994).